Strength-Boosting Superfoods

Fuelling Your Fitness Fire

Table of Contents

Chapter 1. Introduction

Unleash the power within you by igniting your fitness regime with the fuel of strength-boosting superfoods. In this Special Report, we unveil the secrets behind the foods that not only nourish your body but also enhance your strength. If you're pursuing a fit and vigorous lifestyle, then this enlightening guide is your golden ticket. We've dug deep, debunked myths, and separated fact from fiction to cherry-pick nature's top powerhouses that are essential for turning your body into a fortress of strength. Each page spills with insights and tips that are as delicious as the foods we're touting! So, throw your fitness hat on and prepare for a joyride of healthy eating and strength-boosting discoveries that will send you sprinting down Body-Boost Boulevard, no looking back. Let's get fueled up! Join us, dive in, and embrace the energy that these superfoods bring. It's time to fan your fitness fire!

Chapter 2. Strength Through Nutrition: The Building Blocks

Eating for fitness isn't just about shedding those extra pounds or achieving that coveted lean physique. It's about becoming robust and enhancing your body's strength from within. To get you started on this rewarding journey, we delve into the fundamentals of nutrition that are key to building strength and vitality.

2.1. Proteins: The Keystone of Strength

You've probably heard it a million times, but here's one more for the record, protein is the building block of life. From cells to tissues to organs, protein takes center stage. It's also an impressive performer in building and repairing muscles. When you're pushing your physical boundaries, whether that's lifting weights, running marathons, or challenging brisk walks, your muscles go through a form of stress, and they need to be repaired with the help of protein.

Incorporate ample high-quality protein in your diet. Chicken breast, lean beef, fish, eggs, tofu, and chickpeas make the table when protein is on the menu. It is recommended that per kilogram of body weight, you consume 1g to 1.5g of protein daily if you're aiming for moderate muscle repair. But if you're after substantial muscle growth, this number should be closer to 2g per kilogram of body weight.

2.2. Carbohydrates: Your Trusted Energy Reserves

Many fitness enthusiasts tend to keep carbohydrates at bay due to a misconstrued apprehension about weight gain. While it's true that inappropriate carbohydrate consumption can lead to undesired body weight, the right type and quantity can dramatically enhance your stamina and strength.

Complex carbohydrates like brown rice, whole grains, sweet potatoes, and oatmeal provide a steady flow of energy that fuels your workouts and aids recovery. Often called slow releasing carbs, they keep your blood glucose levels steady while preventing fat storage.

Do remember that carb consumption should be tailored based on your physical activity. Consuming more carbs than you can burn will undoubtedly lead to weight gain. Healthy adult women and men should aim to consume between 130g and 175g of carbohydrates per day.

2.3. Fats: The Underdog Powerhouse

For decades, fat was vilified as the dietary bad guy. However, science has shown us that not all fats are enemies. Healthy fats, or unsaturated fats, are prized players in cellular health and metabolism. They also act as a backup energy source when carbohydrates are not available.

Monounsaturated and polyunsaturated fats, found in foods such as avocados, nuts, seeds, and fish, should make up a substantial portion of your fat intake. On a 2,000-calorie daily diet, about 25-30% of your calorie intake should come from fats.

2.4. Vitamins and Minerals: Your Inner Defense League

Vitamins and minerals might not directly influence your muscle mass or strength, but they are critical in facilitating the function and maintenance of your body. For instance, Vitamin D aids in calcium absorption, essential for bone health and thus indirectly contributing to strength training. Likewise, Iron helps transport oxygen - a fuel source for your muscles - throughout your body.

Fruits and vegetables are your best friends when it comes to ensuring an ample supply of essential vitamins and minerals. Also, do not underestimate the power of the sun. Just 10-30 minutes of midday sunlight can supply your adequate daily dose of Vitamin D.

2.5. Hydration: Health's Unsung Hero

Water's role in muscle strength might be the less sung tale in the fitness fraternity, but it's no less significant. Water affects nearly every aspect of physical function. Dehydration can swiftly lead to compromised physiological and performance responses during exercise.

Active individuals should drink about 3.7 liters (or about 13 cups) for men and 2.7 liters (about 9 cups) for women per day. Exercise in hot or humid weather can increase your daily water needs.

2.6. Nutrient Timing: The Unsaid Secret

"People who think they have no time for healthy eating will sooner or later have to find time for illness." - Edward Stanley.

Nutrient timing, simply put, is consuming specific nutrients such as protein or carbohydrates at certain times for optimal benefit. For instance, consuming protein post-workout aids muscle recovery and growth, whereas a pre-workout carbohydrate meal can serve as an energy booster.

While individual responses to nutrient timing strategies can vary, it is generally acknowledged that an effective strategy can lend a significant hand in accomplishing fitness and strength endurance.

Strength through nutrition is not an elusive concept but a practical, realizable goal. Embrace these fundamentals, experiment with them, and see the difference they make in your journey towards superior strength. The beauty of eating well is that it feels good. The even greater joy is that good eating gives you the strength to live your life the way you want — to its fullest.

Chapter 3. Unmasking the Superfoods: A Deeper Look

Superfoods have risen to fame in the health and fitness world due to their nutrient-dense profiles. Participants of the fit lifestyle movement have started recognizing these foods for their ability to enhance physical strength and overall well-being.

3.1. What Are Superfoods?

Superfoods aren't your everyday food items, they are fruits, vegetables, grains, and proteins that have exceptionally high nutritive value. They are rich in vitamins, minerals, antioxidants, fiber, and other essential nutrients, all of which contribute to building and maintaining a strong, hearty body. The term 'superfood' isn't an official classification rather, a marketing term adopted to describe these nutritional powerhouses.

3.2. Crucial Superfoods for Strength Enhancement

3.3. Quinoa

Quinoa is often hailed as a super grain, even though it's technically a seed. It's rich in complete proteins, providing all the nine essential amino acids our body can't synthesize. This makes it an excellent choice for muscle building and repair after arduous workout sessions.

3.4. Blueberries

Blueberries are tiny fruits packed with antioxidant power. They're abundant in vitamins C and K, which are important for quick muscle recovery. Blueberries also contain a wealth of polyphenols that combat oxidative stress caused by intense exercise.

3.5. Spinach

This leafy green powerhouse brings to mind the legendary strength of the sailor-man, Popeye. And truth be told, there's science behind the cartoon lore. Spinach is rich in iron which is vital for muscle function, and in nitrates, which can promote efficient muscle contraction.

3.6. Almonds

These nuts are rich in Vitamin E, an antioxidant that hunts free radicals fabricated during tough physical activities. They're also a great source of protein and healthy fats– helping with muscle repair and providing slow-release energy.

3.7. Omega-3 Rich Fish

Fish like salmon, trout, and mackerel are loaded with essential Omega-3 fatty acids playing an integral role in cardiovascular health, brain function, and inflammation reduction.

3.8. Milestones in Superfood Research

Since the early 2000s, the scientific community has taken a keen interest in studying the potential health benefits of superfoods. Many studies indicate their crucial role in boosting physical and mental health, as well as preventing chronic diseases. It's of paramount importance to remember that superfoods are not magic bullets, but rather, vital constituents of a balanced diet.

3.9. Superfoods, Exercise, and Strength

While exercising and regular workouts sculpt the body, superfoods provide the necessary fuel. Regular consumption of these nutrient-dense foods augments strength, enhances muscular function, and accelerates recovery. Foods like quinoa, almonds and spinach provide the building blocks for muscle repair and regeneration, while blueberries and other antioxidant-rich foods minimize exercise-induced oxidative stress.

3.10. The Superfood Health Spectrum

The potency of superfoods extends beyond boosting physical strength and enhancing exercise performance. These nutrient-dense foods proffer an array of health benefits from promoting heart health, enhancing immune responses, to supporting mental wellbeing. It is also essential to understand that the consumption of superfoods should complement a balanced meal plan featuring diverse food groups.

3.11. The Power of Superfoods: Perception vs. Reality

Despite the widespread belief in the power of superfoods, it's important to remember that these foods can't offset an otherwise unhealthy diet or lifestyle. No single food, no matter how super, can secure health and well-being in isolation. The consumption of these nutrient-dense foods should synergize with an active lifestyle for optimal results.

3.12. How to Incorporate Superfoods into Your Diet?

The beauty of superfoods lies in their versatility. Simple ways to incorporate these into your diet include adding spinach to your salads or smoothies, swapping meat or poultry with quinoa in meals, and sprinkling almonds or blueberries over your breakfast porridge.

3.13. Be Critical, Yet Open

As with all flashy terms in the health and wellness industry, the term 'superfood' might sometimes be used to sell you expensive and exotic items. Many of the superfoods are simply robust versions of regular food, and you don't necessarily need to invest hugely in foreign alternatives when local produce can often offer similar advantages. Remember, the hallmark of a healthy diet is variety, and this certainly applies to superfoods too.

So yes, superfoods are an essential component of the strength-booster diet. However, it's your job to ensure that they're working in harmony with a balanced diet and an active lifestyle to help you achieve your strength and fitness goals. After all, the road to ultimate strength is a journey, complete with diverse and synergistic dietary and lifestyle choices.

Chapter 4. Power Proteins: Meat-based Strength Foods

Exploring the world of strength-boosting foods, one cannot discount the importance of protein. The building block of our muscles, protein plays a pivotal role in building strength, repairing tissues, and maintaining a well-functioning immune system. This chapter will focus on meat-based proteins that are renowned for their strength-enhancing properties.

4.1. The Unyielding Power of Protein

Protein is vital for the human body, and it takes center stage when it comes to muscle building and repair. Comprised of amino acids, protein is the primary element in the construction and repair of tissues, including muscles. When you exercise or perform any strenuous activity, the muscle tissue faces microscopic damage. The body uses protein to repair these micro-tears and thus builds stronger, larger muscles.

Meat, the classic protein source, can be particularly beneficial because it's a complete protein, meaning it contains all nine essential amino acids needed for the body to function. This makes meat a powerhouse for strength training and hence an essential element in our power protein exploration.

4.2. Chicken: The Lean Protein staple

Chicken, particularly the chicken breast, is a staple ingredient in any fitness enthusiast's diet. Chicken breast provides about 31 grams of protein per 100 grams, making it one of the most protein-dense foods available.

However, it's not only about the massive protein punch that chicken packs. It also offers a rich supply of vitamins B6, B12, niacin (B3), and choline, all of which play an integral part in optimizing bodily functions.

4.3. Turkey: Leaner and Meaner

Along with chicken, turkey features prominently on the list of good protein sources. Lean turkey meat is low in fat and high in protein, containing an impressive 29 grams per 100 grams. Just like chicken, turkey meat is also packed with vitamins B6, B12, niacin, and choline.

Besides, turkey meat also includes selenium, an essential mineral that contributes to thyroid hormone metabolism, reproduction, DNA synthesis, and protection from oxidative damage and infection.

4.4. Red Meat: Fuel for the Powerhouse

For those who aren't shy about their love for red meat, you likely know the joy and flavor that comes with it. But did you know that red meat is a complete protein packed with extra nutrients like iron, zinc, and vitamin B12?

Beef, for instance, boasts about 26 grams of protein per 100 grams. However, it's essential to be mindful of the cuts of meat. Opting for lean cuts can help manage your fat intake while providing you with the protein boost you need for strength gains.

4.5. Fish: The Omega-3 Filled Protein Source

When discussing a strength-enhancing diet, we usually imagine chicken, beef, or turkey. However, fish is a powerful contender in this race, supplying a hefty amount of protein and a smattering of vitamins and minerals.

Fish like salmon, rich in protein (20 grams per 100 grams) and packed with omega-3 fatty acids, is not just about muscle building but also about maintaining excellent overall health. Omega-3 fatty acids help reduce inflammation, support mental health, and contribute to heart health, making fish a well-rounded protein source.

4.6. Pork: The Protein-Rich White Meat

Often overlooked, pork is an excellent source of meat-based protein that is as versatile in cooking as chicken. With about 27 grams of protein per 100 grams, pork is up there with the other protein giants. It's also a good source of thiamine, selenium, and zinc, making it a robust choice for strength and overall wellness.

Remember, while it's easy to focus solely on the protein content of food, keeping a balanced diet that incorporates a great variety of nutrients should always be the goal. After all, turning your body into a fortress of strength isn't just about protein. It's about taking care of every aspect of your nutrition.

Meat-based proteins are an excellent choice for many, providing not only high-quality protein but also an abundance of other vitamins and minerals. By intelligently incorporating these into your diet, you can fuel your body optimally for the strength-based journey you're embarking on. So, choose wisely, eat well, and let your strength soar high on the wings of these powerful proteins!

Chapter 5. Plant Power: Vegan Sources of Fitness Fuel

When contemplating the strength and power that can be achieved through a balanced diet, our minds might instantly gravitate towards images of carnivorous bodybuilders and athletes. However, the power of plants in achieving, and even surpassing, these same fitness goals cannot be underestimated. In this chapter, we're going to expand our horizons and explore the plethora of vegan-friendly foods that pack a punch in the fitness arena and how they can be integrated into your regimen to amplify your strength and stamina.

5.1. The Protein Powerhouses

Proteins fundamentally serve as the building blocks of our bodies. They are crucial for building and repairing tissues, including muscles, and enabling growth. Invariably, they are a prerequisite for any fitness-oriented diet.

Though animal products are often credited with being protein-rich, numerous plants offer substantial amounts of this essential nutrient. For strength and fitness seekers adhering to a vegan diet, the following stand out:

1. Soy: Tofu, tempeh, and edamame all originate from soybeans. Soy is a complete protein, meaning it contains all nine essential amino acids your body needs.

2. Quinoa: Another complete protein, quinoa, is a grain that's not only high in protein but also rich in fiber and minerals.

3. Lentils: Just one cup of cooked lentils provides 18 grams of protein. They're also a great source of slowly digested carbs, and a full meal combined with rice or bread.

4. Beans and Chickpeas: Apart from being high in protein, they're

also rich in complex carbs, fiber, iron, folate, phosphorus, potassium, manganese, and several beneficial plant compounds.

5. Seitan: Made from gluten, the main protein in wheat, seitan is a popular protein source for many vegetarians and vegans. It's also a good source of selenium and contains small amounts of iron, calcium, and phosphorus.

5.2. The Carb Code

Carbohydrates form the next piece of the puzzle. They provide the energy required by the body during workouts. Vegan diets typically abound in carbohydrates, and the key is to harness these foods for their slow-release energy.

Integrating whole, unrefined carbohydrates into your meals and snacks will ensure steady energy release, limit peaks and troughs in blood sugars, and help maintain optimal performance. Excellent vegan sources include sweet potatoes, brown rice, oats, bananas, black beans, and lentils.

5.3. Vegan Fat Facts

Healthy fats play a significant role in a fitness diet. They aid the absorption of nutrients, produce necessary hormones, and provide long-lasting energy. As a vegan, you can obtain healthy fats from a variety of plant foods:

1. Avocados: Besides being an excellent source of healthy fats, they contain a plethora of vitamins and minerals.

2. Chia Seeds: These seeds are an incredible source of omega-3 fatty acids, antioxidants, fiber, iron, and calcium.

3. Flaxseeds: Flaxseeds are processed by the body to make omega-3 fatty acids. They're also an excellent source of dietary fiber.

4. Nuts and Nut Butters: Almonds, cashews, and peanuts are a wonderful vegan source of healthy fats and protein.

5.4. Essential Vitamins and Minerals

To ensure you are getting a broad spectrum of vitamins and minerals, it's important to consume a variety of fruits, vegetables, grains, and legumes. Leafy greens, berries, sweet potatoes, apples, bananas, quinoa, brown rice, lentils, and chickpeas provide a wealth of vitamins and minerals essential for fitness.

5.5. Superfood Smoothies

Smoothies offer a fantastic, easily digested way to pack a host of fitness fuels into one meal. Think of combining a variety of what we've mentioned above to keep you filled and fueled for a longer time. For example, a high-protein smoothie might include spinach, hemp seeds, chia seeds, almond butter, and a handful of blueberries. The options are limitless!

With the right choice and combination of these plant-based foods, any fitness aficionado can not only meet their dietary needs but truly thrive. Remember, variety is the spice of, not only life but a nutritious diet too! Combining various plant-based sources will ensure a complete nutritional profile, supporting your body's strength and endurance goals with gusto. So, get ready to harness the power of plants and let vegan fitness fuel propel your journey towards peak fitness.

Chapter 6. Supercharged Seafood: Oceans of Energy

Crashing waves, dynamic life, and an awe-inspiring tapestry of biodiversity—the ocean is not just a vast source of inspiration but a cornucopia of nourishment too. From its deep trenches to its sparkling surface, it thrives with life that fuels our health, fitness, and overall well-being. It's high time we shine a spotlight on the unique power of seafood—a grand symphony of nutritional gems, exotic flavors, and amazing health benefits that help you achieve an enhanced state of physical strength and vigor.

6.1. The Nutritional Power Punch: A Deep Dive

When it comes to using the term 'superfood,' there are few items as deserving of this title as seafood. Packed with essential nutrients while low in saturated fats, seafood is a potent source of lean protein that fuels muscle growth and recovery.

High-quality protein provided by seafood dishes bolsters your body in fitness training, healing any microscopic muscle tears caused by intense workouts. It's not just the protein, but also the unique blend of amino acids present in seafood that facilitates the muscle recovery process. Think of these amino acids as the building blocks to a stronger, more resilient body infrastructure.

Seafood also contains a rich dose of omega-3 fatty acids, a powerful nutrient that's not naturally produced by the human body. Omega-3s can help reduce inflammation, lower blood pressure, improve heart health, and even boost brain function. The docosahexaenoic acid (DHA) and eicosapentaenoic acid (EPA), types of omega-3 fatty acids largely found in fatty fish, are crucial for maintaining body strength and sustaining a steady fitness drive.

6.2. Fishy Fitness Stars: Five High-Performing Seafood

Let's delve deeper into the aqueous world to discover some of these supercharged seafood stars teeming with fitness-friendly nutrients.

6.2.1. Salmon: More than Just Omega-3

Salmon is renowned for its unparalleled high omega-3 content, but there's more to this aquatic superstar. It's also a prominent source of high-quality protein, vitamins B12 and D, selenium, and niacin. Salmon's impressive nutritional profile makes it a compelling choice to fuel your workouts and foster a robust immunity.

6.2.2. Tuna: The Lean Machine

Tuna, besides being a lean source of high-quality protein, is packed with essential nutrients like Vitamin B complex, selenium, and magnesium. Fresh tuna also has a respectable dose of heart-healthy omega-3 fatty acids. Consider incorporating this strong-swimming species into your diet for a wholesome blend of nutrients that'll endure through the toughest workouts.

6.2.3. Shellfish: The Nutrient-Dense Delicacies

Clams, mussels, oysters, and scallops offer a substantial amount of lean protein along with a cocktail of other nutrients like Vitamin B12, iron, and zinc. Oysters, in particular, are a rich dietary source of zinc, a mineral linked to improved immunity and muscle growth.

6.2.4. Sardines: The Small but Mighty

Despite their small size, sardines pack a hefty nutritional punch. Loaded with omega-3 fatty acids, these little fishes also bring essential nutrients like Vitamin D, calcium, and selenium to your platter. They're especially advantageous for people looking to build bone strength alongside muscle fortification.

6.2.5. Halibut: The Silent Powerhouse

Halibut, a less-talked-about fish, boasts impressive nutritional stats. It's not only a hulk in terms of protein content, but also a prime source of magnesium, selenium, phosphorus, zinc, and Vitamins B6, B12, and D. Incorporating halibut into your fitness nutrition regime can assist in strengthening your body from inside out.

6.3. The Sea-to-Table Voyage: Choosing and Preparing Seafood

Choosing the right fish and shellfish is a crucial part of the journey. Aim for fresh, wild-caught options whenever possible. However, frozen seafood can also be a fantastic choice, retaining most of the nutrient profile while offering convenience in modern hectic routines.

Preparing seafood mindfully matters too. Opt for cooking methods like grilling, steaming, baking or boiling to maintain the nutritive value. Overcooking can degrade the omega-3 content and lead to nutrient loss, thus make sure you follow precise cooking times. And remember, it's always best to sidestep fried seafood or dishes laden with heavy cream sauces to avoid unnecessary fats and calories.

6.4. Understanding Seafood Sustainability

In the pursuit of health and fitness, we cannot ignore our responsibility towards the environment and the preservation of the marine ecosystem. Choosing sustainably sourced seafood can play a significant role in this endeavor. Look for certifications like Marine Stewardship Council (MSC) or Aquaculture Stewardship Council (ASC) to ensure you're supporting responsible fishing and farming practices.

Marine potency should not be undervalued in the realm of fitness. Embracing the gifts of oceans and incorporating them into your dietary regime opens up new avenues of strength, fitness, and overall health. It's not just about having a physical edge; it's also about instilling a sense of discipline, knowing that what you choose to consume contributes to your progress, vitality, and resilience. So, are you ready to dive into the deep blue world of supercharged seafood? It's time to cast the net and reel in your strength-enriching catch!

Chapter 7. Super Fruits and Super Vegetables: Nature's Candy

Every fitness journey is an intricate interplay of mindful exercise, rest, and a healthy diet. A cornerstone of the latter is the incredible variety and bounty of fruits and vegetables. These everyday foods up the ante when it comes to delivering explosive bursts of energy while packing a nutritive punch. In this extensive discussion, we dissect the health benefits and ways to incorporate nature's candies - the super fruits and super vegetables - into one's eating habits, to help realize a fit and firm physique.

7.1. Super Fruits: Juicy Bombs of Power

Super fruits are a gamut of fruits overflowing with a luxurious supply of vitamins, minerals, and antioxidants. The high concentration of these essential nutrients can support the body's energy levels, protect against disease, and aid in recovery and growth.

1. **Bananas:** Packed with essential carbohydrates, bananas are the perfect energy boosters pre-workout. They are rich in potassium that helps manage muscle contractions and potassium losses during workouts. A natural energy bar, bananas are the ideal on-the-go snack for athletes and fitness enthusiasts alike.

2. **Berries:** Blueberries, strawberries, raspberries, and blackberries are loaded with antioxidants, fiber, and vitamin C. These little marvels can help neutralize harmful free radicals, aid digestion, and bolster immune function. Throw a handful into your protein

shake for a nutrient-packed breakfast.

3. **Avocados:** While technically a fruit, avocados have a unique nutritional profile with a high amount of monounsaturated fats that can aid in nutrient absorption. Rich in vitamin E, avocados help reduce inflammation, perfect for post-workout muscle recovery.

7.2. Super Vegetables: Green Machines of Health

Like their fruity counterparts, super vegetables offer a powerhouse of nutrients and health benefits. Green leafy vegetables, cruciferous veg, and others provide dietary fiber, loads of vitamins, and a helping of major minerals.

1. **Spinach:** This green leafy vegetable is overflowing with nutrients like iron, calcium, and magnesium. The high iron content aids in oxygen transportation to the muscles, key for cellular energy production.

2. **Broccoli:** A member of the cruciferous vegetable family, broccoli is dense with a variety of vitamins, fiber, and potent antioxidants like sulforaphane. Regular consumption of this super vegetable can decrease oxidative stress and boost heart health.

3. **Sweet Potatoes:** A staple for any fitness-minded individual, sweet potatoes are loaded with vitamin A, potassium, and slow-digesting carbohydrates. They help maintain energy levels and support muscle recovery. Include them post-workout for best results.

7.3. Incorporating Super Fruits and Vegetables into Your Diet

Ensuring these superfoods are a part of your daily intake can significantly boost your fitness journey. Here are some tasty and easy ways to incorporate them into your routine.

1. **Breakfast Smoothies:** Blend fruits like berries, bananas, and a handful of spinach to create a nutrient-dense smoothie. Add a scoop of your favorite protein powder for an extra protein punch.

2. **Salads and Sautéed Veggies:** Leafy salads with a variety of colorful vegetables not only satiate hunger but ensure a nutrient-dense meal. Additionally, lightly sautéing vegetables like broccoli can make for a delicious and healthy side dish.

3. **Snacks and Desserts:** Choose fruits for snacking over unhealthy chips or cookies. Use dates or figs to sweeten desserts, making them a healthier indulgence.

These are just some of the ways super fruits and vegetables can strengthen and fuel your body, but the possibilities are endless. Remember, the path to robust health and a fit body is an exciting culinary journey rather than a punishing regime. So, get creative, and enjoy the flavors of health and fitness!

In conclusion, nature's candy, super fruits, and super vegetables, power packed with essential nutrients, can play a pivotal role in your fitness journey. Coupled with appropriate physical activity, these foods can amplify your strength, enhance healing, and reinforce your resilience. So, here's to embarking on a nutritious journey down the path of supreme health and unbounded fitness! Enjoy the ride and keep those muscles pumping!

Chapter 8. Nuts and Seeds: Small Size, Big Impact

When it comes to packing a nutritional punch in bite-sized packages, nuts and seeds take the crown. But what exactly is it that makes these tiny titans perfect for enhancing strength balanced with overall wellness? We'll uncover it all, step by step.

8.1. Meet Your Nutrient Powerhouses

Nuts and seeds, both minuscule in size, might seem like an unlikely source of energy. However, their nutrient profile is anything but small.

Known primarily for their substantial content of healthy fats, nuts, and seeds also flaunt impressive quantities of proteins, antioxidants, vitamins, and minerals – all in a compact package. The fats in nuts are primarily monounsaturated fats, along with notable amounts of omega-3 and omega-6 fatty acids, which are all heart-healthy. Seeds also boast a good composition of beneficial fatty acids, though the types and proportions can vary depending on the seed variety.

The protein content in nuts and seeds is valuable for building and repairing body tissues, including muscles. This makes them an excellent food option for strength training. A 30 g serving of almonds, for example, delivers around 6 grams of protein. The protein content in seeds can vary more widely, though certain ones, like chia seeds, are known for their relatively high protein content.

Vitamins and minerals dot the landscape of nuts and seeds as well. They're rich in Vitamin E, a potent antioxidant that protects your cells from damage, and several B Vitamins, which play a critical role in energy metabolism. Minerals like magnesium, phosphorus, and zinc are abundantly present, each one playing a vital role in muscle function, energy production, and immunity.

8.2. Variety Matters: The Strength Secrets of Different Nuts and Seeds

While all nuts and seeds make a worthwhile contribution to a strength-boosting diet, different varieties shine in unique aspects:

- **Almonds**: Packed with proteins, antioxidant-rich Vitamin E, and bone-booster calcium, almonds champion the cause of muscle function and recovery.

- **Walnuts**: Walnuts are famous for their omega-3 fatty acid content, which aid in reducing inflammation resulting from strenuous workouts.

- **Peanuts**: Despite being technically legumes, peanuts exhibit the characteristics of nuts when it comes to nutritional profile. They stand out for their protein content and heart-healthy monounsaturated fats.

- **Flaxseeds**: These seeds are a rich source of alpha-linolenic acid, a type of omega-3 fat, and lignans, compounds that could protect against heart disease and some types of cancers.

- **Chia Seeds**: These tiny black seeds pack a high fiber punch desiringly delaying gastric emptying, meaning prolonged nutrient absorption. They're also an excellent source of plant-based omega-3s and can gel when mixed with liquid, making them a great ingredient option for energy gels.

8.3. Incorporating Nuts and Seeds into Your Fitness Diet

It's clear that adding nuts and seeds to your diet can ramp up your fitness game, but how exactly should you integrate these powerhouses into your meals?

One of the most straightforward ways is to snack on a handful of nuts between meals. They're filling, satisfying, and easy to carry, making them a perfect on-the-go option.

If you're a smoothie enthusiast, adding a tablespoon or two of your chosen nuts or seeds can instantly boost the protein content of your drink, making it an excellent post-workout recovery option. If you lean towards oatmeal or yogurt for breakfast, sprinkle some nuts and seeds on top for a welcome crunch and a nutrient kick.

Nuts and seeds also make a delicious addition to salads, giving them a boost both in terms of texture and nutritional value. Or, they can be ground into a flour and added to protein pancakes or baked goods, further enhancing the protein content and providing necessary healthy fats.

An exciting way to include seeds, specifically chia or flax, is by using them as an egg substitute in recipes if you're looking for a vegan option. Mix one tablespoon of flaxseed meal or chia seeds with two and a half tablespoons of water and let it sit for about 5 minutes to gel, creating what's known as a "flax egg" or "chia egg."

8.4. Protein-Packed Recipes Using Nuts and Seeds

Looking for culinary inspiration to incorporate these nutrient-dense foods into your regular diet? Here are two delicious, simple recipes you can try:

1. **Almond Joy Protein Shake**

2. **Chia Seed Protein Bars**

Nuts and Seeds: Power in Moderation

Despite their nutrient density, nuts and seeds are also high in calories, so practicing portion control is essential. It's recommended to stick to a one-ounce serving of nuts (about a handful) or a tablespoon or two of seeds to get the nutritional benefits without overdoing it on calories.

Choosing raw or dry-roasted versions without added salt will provide you most benefits. Soaking and sprouting nuts and seeds can also increase digestibility and the availability of some nutrients.

In summary, don't let their size fool you. These small soldiers are ready to energize your strength routine and nourish your body at the same time. Include them in your diet, savor the taste, and embrace the fitness benefits that come along the journey. Nuts and seeds truly confirm the saying- "Good things come in small packages."

Chapter 9. Whole Grains: The Slow-Burning Fuels

Whole grains are the essential treasure troves of slow-releasing energy and the cornerstone of an optimal fitness diet. Often underestimated in the world of trendy "low-carb", "keto" and "paleo" diets, whole grains can play a crucial role in keeping the body fueled and fortified for high-strength activities. They are nature's multivitamins and wonders of natural packaging that comprise bran, germ, and endosperm, providing a bombshell of vitamins, minerals, fiber, and protein.

9.1. A Closer Look at What Whole Grains Are

Whole grains, or foods made from them, contain all essential parts and naturally occurring nutrients of the entire grain seed in their original proportions. The grain has three main parts: the bran, the germ, and the endosperm. The bran, or the outer skin, is packed to the brim with an impressive lineup of fiber, antioxidants and B-vitamins, while the germ is no slacker with a concentrated dose of vitamins E and B, phytochemicals, antioxidants and healthy fats. The endosperm, the largest part of the seed, brings up the rear with starch and a bit of protein and vitamins. The intricate synergy of all these components makes whole grains a nutritive reservoir of slow-burning fuel for your body.

9.2. Delving into the Nutritional Profiling of Whole Grains

Each type of whole grain brings a unique mix of nutrients to the table, ensuring that they cater to a wide array of your metabolic needs. A rich source of carbohydrates, whole grains provide long-lasting energy that helps maintain your body's fuel during intense workouts.

A prominent part of their nutritional profile is their substantial reservoir of dietary fiber. Fiber is vital for a healthy gut, an essential companion for anyone pursuing a healthy lifestyle. These high-fiber allies aid in digestion, support weight management, and maintain cardiac health by reducing harmful LDL cholesterol concentrations. They also keep blood sugar levels steady, preventing sharp spikes and plunges.

As for vitamins and minerals, they're no strangers to whole grains either. They're packed with B-vitamins – thiamin (B1), riboflavin (B2), and niacin (B3), which are critical in energy production and cell function. They also contain minerals such as iron, which is essential in oxygen transportation in the blood, magnesium for bone health and hundreds of biochemical reactions, and selenium, a potent antioxidant.

Along with this, they have protein, the fundamental building block for muscles and tissues. Evidently, whole grains are a superior source for all-round nourishment of your body.

9.3. The Health Power-Punch Whole Grains Deliver

Whole grains do more than just energy provision; they render various health benefits that make them a must-have in your everyday diet. Regular intake of whole grains has shown to reduce the risk of chronic diseases like heart disease, Type 2 diabetes, and certain types of cancer. They play a role in maintaining healthy body weight, reducing inflammation, and promoting gut health.

9.4. Understanding the Glycemic Impact

Whole grains have a low to medium glycemic index, meaning the carbohydrates present in them gradually break down into glucose and get absorbed into the bloodstream. This slow release of glucose provides a steady energy supply, fuels brain function, and maintains a steady metabolic rate. It keeps you full for longer, preventing unnecessary snacking and aiding weight control.

9.5. The List of Fitness-Friendly Whole Grains

Whole Grain	Benefits	Best way to incorporate
Oats	Rich in beta-glucan fiber. Lower LDL cholesterol.	Protein-packed oatmeal for breakfast.
Brown Rice	Excellent source of essential minerals.	A bowl of brown rice with veggies for lunch.
Quinoa	Complete protein grain. Filled with antioxidants.	Add quinoa to salads or have it as a side dish.
Buckwheat	Rich in protein and fiber. Gluten-free.	Use as a cereal or in baked goods.
Barley	Rich in fiber. Benefits digestion.	Make barley soup or stew.
Whole Wheat	High Fiber. Prevents constipation.	Whole wheat bread for sandwich.

Whole grains come in many varieties and flavors, making them a compatible constituent to any meal of the day. They provide your body with sustained energy to bolster fitness and strength.

9.6. Turning the Tide on Popular Misconceptions

Despite their profound benefits, whole grains often get sidelined. One misconception is that grains lead to weight gain due to their carbohydrate content. But when paired with regular physical activity, the carbohydrates in whole grains provide the necessary fuel for your body. Another common misconception is that all grains are equal - refined grains don't hold a candle to 'whole' grains when it comes to nutrient composition, fiber content, or any health benefits.

9.7. The Ultimate Verdict

Whole grains are the quintessential component of a strength-boosting fitness diet. They provide not only an abundant amount of energy but also a profusion of nutrients and health benefits that amplify overall wellbeing. Heavy on nutrients and light on the digestive system, they muster both taste and health, making them an absolute win-win. Commit to the wholesome regimen of including whole grains in your diet, and savor the strength that they bring to your fitness game.

Chapter 10. Hydration Station: Fluids That Energize

If there's ever a magic potion that fuels our bodies, it's water. This seemingly simple life-giver holds the power to invigorate the body, mind, and soul. It hydrates and rejuvenates us, flushing out toxins, and transporting nutrients to where they're needed most. But do you know what's more exciting? The delicious hydrating drinks that not only refresh us but also load us with nutrients for a strength-boosting punch. Let's dive right into the ocean of fluids that energize.

10.1. The crown holder: Water

It can't be emphasized enough - good old H2O is paramount. Water is involved in nearly every body function, from aiding digestion to maintaining temperature and transporting nutrients. It's essential for a myriad of biochemical reactions, and even a slight drop in hydration levels can impact physical and cognitive performance. Adults should aim for about 2-3 liters of fluids daily - but remember that individual needs may vary based on factors like activity levels, climate, and diet.

10.2. Energy in a cup: Hydrating Herbal Teas

Delving into the world of energizing fluids, you cannot miss the wonder that is herbal teas. Whether it's a steaming cup of peppermint tea to revitalize your senses or chamomile tea for deep relaxation - herbal teas are little nutrient-packed powerhouses. They hydrate, provide essential antioxidants, and come with their unique health benefits, boosting your strength from inside out. There's indeed a tea for every mood and requirement, ensuring you're spoilt for choice.

10.3. Nectar of Strength: Natural Fruit Juices

Reaching out for a glass of fruit juice provides instant hydration and an impactful dose of vitamins, antioxidants, and other beneficial compounds. However, it's important to ensure that juices are freshly squeezed and consumed rather than opting for the processed versions laden with sugars and preservatives. Better still, make sure to include the pulp that's full of dietary fiber. Remember, while juices are nutritious, they should not replace whole fruits in the diet but should complement them.

10.4. Go Nuts Over Coconut Water

Brimming with vitamins, minerals, and electrolytes, coconut water can serve as a powerful natural sports drink. It is particularly rich in potassium, which helps balance electrolytes, regulate muscle function, and manage water balance. With its fresh, lightly sweet taste, coconut water not only hydrates but also makes for an energizing, refreshing treat.

10.5. All hail the power of Green Tea

Caffeinated drinks, when consumed within limits, can provide an instant energy boost. Among them, green tea holds a special place. Packed with antioxidants and tannins, it offers a gentle, sustainable energy boost without leading to the "crash" associated with stronger caffeinated drinks. And it's not just about energy - the catechins in green tea have been linked to a range of health benefits, making it a healthy choice.

10.6. Milk: A powerhouse of nutrition

Often overlooked in discussions of hydrating drinks, milk is actually about 90% water and packed with valuable nutrients like calcium, protein, B vitamins, and minerals. Chocolate milk has gained a reputation as an effective recovery drink post-exercise due to its optimal carbohydrate and protein content.

10.7. Super Smoothies for the Win

Vibrant smoothies made from a blend of fruits, greens, nuts, seeds, milk, or yogurt offer more than just tantalizing taste experiences. Along with hydration, they deliver a hearty dose of fibers, healthy fats, proteins, and numerous vitamins and minerals. They are excellent for a post-workout recharge or a nutrient-rich snack to fuel your strength-based lifestyle.

10.8. Kombucha: The fermented marvel

While being an excellent hydrating option, kombucha also tops the chart in promoting gut health. This fizzy, tangy drink is packed with probiotics (healthy bacteria) that can aid digestion and immunity. Apart from hydration and nutrition, healthy gut flora plays a significant role in overall strength and wellness.

Life thrives on hydration, and these fluids not only do the job but bring along an excellent bundle of nutrients to power up your strength levels. So, drink up and keep the fitness fire burning ferociously bright+!

Chapter 11. Recipes for Strength: Whipping Up Fitness Foods in Your Kitchen

Eating healthy is integral to fueling your fitness journey and gaining strength. There's no denying that a carefully crafted, nutrient-rich diet can deliver strong, noticeable results when coupled with a diligent exercise regimen. Today, let's dive into the heart of your kitchen, the ultimate location where strength-building begins. If you're geared up to transform your meals into power-packed supplements of vigorous health, then let's get started!

11.1. The Superfood Power Trio

When it comes to striking the ideal balance between taste and nutrition, three key pillars come to play- proteins, carbohydrates, and fats - the classic power trio! Bringing together these nutrients at the heart of your meals does not merely add flavor; it fuels your body with the essential elements it needs to boost strength and resilience.

- **Proteins:** Crucial for repairing and building tissues, proteins are the building blocks that our body utilizes to heal after strenuous workouts. They assist in muscle development, providing a strong base for our physical strength. Examples of protein-rich foods include eggs, lean meats, yogurt, cheese, and a variety of legumes.

- **Carbohydrates:** Contrary to popular belief, carbs are not your enemy. They're our body's primary source of energy. Foods rich in carbohydrates help restore glycogen levels and promote recovery after intense workouts. Excellence sources include whole grains, fruits, vegetables, and legumes.

- **Fats:** It's time to debunk the myth that 'all fats are bad'. Healthy fats fuel your body, aid in the absorption of vitamins, and help maintain core body temperature. Food sources like avocado, olive oil, flax seeds, and almonds contain the 'good' fats necessary for maintaining optimal health.

11.2. The Recipe Cookup: Strength Building Meals

Armed with the knowledge of our power trio, the next step is constructing meals centered around these food groups. Let's explore a few recipes that can be quickly whipped up in your kitchen, promising taste and a strength boost.

11.2.1. Bountiful Breakfast: Banana and Nut Smoothie

Kick start your day with a refreshing, protein-packed, and delicious smoothie.

Ingredients:

1. 1 large Banana

2. 1 cup Almond milk

3. 2 tablespoons Peanut butter

4. 1 tablespoon Honey

5. 1/4 cup Greek yogurt

6. 1 tablespoon Chia seeds

Blend everything until smooth, and your power-packed breakfast is ready to consume!

11.2.2. Strength Lunch: Quinoa and Grilled Chicken Salad

Power up your mid-day meals with this easy to make quinoa and chicken salad.

Ingredients:

1. 1 cup Quinoa
2. 2 cups Water
3. 2 Grilled chicken breasts
4. 1 cup Spinach, chopped
5. 1/2 cup Cherry tomatoes
6. 1/2 cup Cucumber, diced
7. 1/4 cup Feta cheese, crumbled

Cook the quinoa in water until it fluffs up. Toss the quinoa along with the veggies, grilled chicken, and feta cheese for a fulfilling and strength enhancing lunch!

11.2.3. Energy Dinner: Baked Salmon with Steamed Vegetables

End your day on a high note with a nutrient-rich dinner.

Ingredients:

1. 2 Salmon fillets
2. 1 tablespoon Olive oil
3. Salt and pepper to taste
4. 1/2 cup Carrots, sliced
5. 1/2 cup Broccoli florets

Marinate the salmon fillets with olive oil, salt, and pepper. Bake at 400°F for 15-20 minutes. Simultaneously, steam your vegetables. Once done, serve the salmon with steamed vegetables. Voila, your balanced dinner is ready!

11.3. Snacking Right: Quick Strength Snacks

Smart snacking can enhance your energy levels and prepare your body for the next workout. Here are a few quick snacks that you can prepare:

- **Trail Mix:** Combine your favorite dried fruits, nuts, and seeds. It's portable and a quick source of energy.

- **Greek Yogurt Parfait:** Layer Greek yogurt, granola, and fruits, and enjoy a protein and carb-rich treat.

- **Hard-Boiled Eggs with Avocado:** A quick, protein-rich snack loaded with healthy fats with a satisfying texture.

No matter what your health and fitness goals may be, the right foods can make all the difference. Harness the power of the superfood power trio, experiment with recipes, and make your own fitness-friendly meals. Remember, your body needs the right fuel, so cook smart and eat smart to sprint towards your fitness goals!